SUPER FOOD GUIDE TO HEALTHY WEIGHT LOSS

by professional health and wellness coach

BRYAN DANIELS

Table Of Contents

Bryan Daniels

Table Of Contents 1

INTRODUCTION 2

SUPER MEAT 3

SUPER VEGGIES 8

SUPER FRUITS 11

SUPER COMPLEX CARBOHYDRATES 14

SUPER DAIRY 16

WHAT ABOUT CALCIUM? 20

CONCLUSION 21

INTRODUCTION

Weight loss and management are excellent ways to extend your life naturally and live a fuller, happier life. While exercise is the best way to trim weight fast, it must go together with proper nutrition. Nutrition is the process of obtaining the food necessary for health and growth. Unfortunately, most people don't know where to begin. Thankfully, we provide top quality nutrition therapy tips to help improve your quality of life!

SUPER MEAT

GRASS-FED BEEF

Protein Payout: 4 oz strip steak, 133 calories, 26 g protein

When it comes to steak or burgers, go grass-fed. It may ding your wallet, but it'll dent your abs. Grass-fed beef is naturally leaner and has fewer calories than conventional meat: A lean seven-ounce conventional strip steak has 386 calories and 16 grams of fat. But a seven-ounce grass-fed strip steak has only 234 calories and five grams of fat. Grass-fed meat according to a study published in Nutrition Journal, is said to contain higher level of omega-3 fatty acids, which have been shown to reduce the risk of heart disease.

BISON

Protein Payout: 4 oz, 166 calories, 23 g of protein

While grass-fed beef is an excellent choice, bison's profile has been rising in recent years, and for a good reason: It has half the fat of and fewer calories than red meat. According to the USDA, while a 90%-lean hamburger may average 10 grams of fat, a comparatively sized buffalo burger rings in at two grams of fat with 24 grams of protein, making it one of the leanest meats around. But wait, taking a chance on this unexpected meat will earn you two healthy bonuses: In just one serving, you'll get a full day's allowance of vitamin B-12, which has been shown to boost energy and help shut down the genes responsible for insulin resistance and the formation of fat cells; additionally, since bison are naturally grass-fed, you can confidently down your burger knowing it's free of the hormones and pollutants than can manifest themselves in your belly fat.

CHICKEN

Protein Payout: 3 oz. cooked breast, 142 calories, 26 g protein

A 3 oz. cooked chicken breast contains only 142 calories and 3 grams of fat, but packs a whopping 26 grams of protein — more than half of the day's recommended allowance. But the go-to protein can be a fail on the taste front. (Our casual poll on the taste of plain breast elicited answers ranging from "air you cut with a knife" to "wet sock.") The good news: With just a little creativity, you can make it a savory post-gym dinner or an impressive date-night meal.

TURKEY

Protein Payout: Quarter-pound turkey burger, 140 calories, 16 g protein

Lean and protein-rich, turkey is no longer an automatic substitute for red meat–this bird deserves props on its own. A quarter-pound turkey burger patty contains 140 calories, 16 grams of protein and eight grams of fat. Additionally, turkey is rich in DHA omega-3 acids—18 mg per serving, the highest on this list—which has been shown to boost brain function, improve your mood and turn off fat genes, preventing fat cells from growing in size. Just make sure you buy white meat only; dark contains too much fat. And know that you're doing your health a double solid by grilling at home: Restaurant versions can be packed with fatty add-ins to increase flavor.

SHELLED PUMPKIN SEEDS

Protein Payout: 1 oz, 158 calories, 9 g protein

Dr. Lindsey Duncan, a nutritionist who has worked with Tony Dorsett and Reggie Bush, is a big fan of pumpkin seeds. "A handful of raw pepitas or dry roasted pumpkin seeds can give you a natural jolt to power through a workout," he says. "They're a good source of protein, healthy fats and fiber, keeping you feeling full and energized longer, and contain manganese, magnesium, phosphorus and zinc, which provide additional energy support to maximize gym time." Throw them into salads and rice dishes or eat them raw.

TEMPEH

Protein Payout: 16 grams per ½ cup

Mas macho than its softer cousin, tofu (which can lead to man boobs), tempeh is made from soy beans, rather than soy milk. As a result, it's closer to a whole food, and keeps more of its protein, about 50% more than tofu.

HALIBUT

Protein Payout: 3 oz, 77 calories, 16 g protein

You already knew fish was rich in protein but you might be surprised to learn that halibut tops fiber-rich oatmeal and vegetables in the satiety department. The Satiety Index of Common Foods, an Australian study published in the European Journal of Clinical Nutrition, ranks it the number two most filling food—bested only by boiled potatoes for its fullness factor. A separate Australian study that compared the satiety of different animal proteins found a nutritionally similar white fish (flake) to be significantly more satiating than beef and chicken; satiety following the white-fish meal also declined at a much slower rate. Study authors attribute the filling factor of white fish like halibut to its impressive protein content and influence on serotonin, one of the key hormones responsible for appetite signals. Just make sure you avoid tilapia.

OSTRICH

Protein Payout: 4 oz patty, 194 calories, 29 g protein

Lower those eyebrows you're raising. Ostrich meat is the rising star of the grill. While it's technically red and has the rich taste of beef, it has less fat than turkey or chicken. A four-ounce patty contains nearly 30 grams of the muscle building nutrient and just six grams of fat. Plus, one serving has 200% of the daily recommended allowance of vitamin B-12. This exotic meat can also help whittle your middle: Ostrich contains 55 milligrams of choline, one of these essential nutrient for fat loss, and it's not as hard to find as it sounds—ostrich is increasingly available in supermarkets around the country.

PORK

Protein Payout: 4 oz, 124 calories, 24 g protein

A longtime enemy of doctors and dieters, pork has been coming around as a healthier alternative of late — as long as you choose the right cut. Your best bet is pork tenderloin: A University of Wisconsin Study found that a three-ounce serving of pork tenderloin has slightly less fat than a skinless chicken breast. It has 24 grams of protein per serving and 83 milligrams of waist-whittling choline (in the latter case, about the same as a medium egg). In a study published in the journal Nutrients, scientists asked 144 overweight people to eat a diet rich in fresh lean pork. After three months, the group saw a significant reduction in waist size, BMI and belly fat, with no reduction in muscle mass! They speculate that the amino acid profile of pork protein may contribute to greater fat burning.

WILD SALMON

Protein Payout: 3 oz, 121 calories, 17 g protein

Don't let salmon's relatively high calorie and fat content fool you; studies suggest the oily fish may be one of the best for weight loss. (In fact, it makes our list of the fatty foods that will help you lose weight.) In one study, participants were divided into groups and assigned one of three equi-caloric weight loss diets that included no seafood (the control group), lean white fish, or salmon. Everyone lost weight, but the salmon eaters had the lowest fasting insulin levels and a marked reduction in inflammation. Another study in the International Journal of Obesity found that eating three 5-ounce servings of salmon per week for four weeks as part of a low-calorie diet resulted in approximately 2.2 pounds more weight lost than following a equip-calorie diet that didn't include fish. Wild salmon is leaner than farmed, which is plumped up on fishmeal; and it's also proven to be significantly lower in cancer-linked PCBs. So go wild — literally.

This is a protein-rich fish you don't want to miss!

LIGHT CANNED TUNA

Protein Payout: 3 oz, 73 calories, 16 g protein

Tuna or to-not? That is the question. As a primo source of protein and docosahexaenoic acid (DHA), canned light tuna is one of the best and most affordable fish for weight loss, especially from your belly! One study in the Journal of Lipid Research showed that omega 3 fatty acid supplementation had the profound ability to turn off abdominal fat genes. And while you'll find two types of fatty acids in cold water fish and fish oils—DHA and eicosapentaenoic acid (EPA)—researchers say DHA can be 40 to 70 percent more effective than EPA at down regulating fat genes in the abdomen, preventing belly fat cells from expanding in size. But what about the mercury? Mercury levels in tuna vary by species; generally speaking, the larger and leaner the fish, the higher the mercury level. Bluefin and albacore rank among the most toxic, according to to a study in Biology Letters. But canned chunk light tuna, harvested from the smallest fish, is considered a "low mercury fish" and can–and should!–be enjoyed two to three times a week (or up to 12 ounces), according to the FDA's most recent guidelines.

SUPER VEGGIES

we admit that's not exactly breaking news, but did you know that when it comes to rapid weight loss some veggies reign supreme while others fall fairly flat in comparison? It's true! Thanks to their specific nutritional profiles, certain produce-aisle picks can help you trim down by revving your metabolism, turning off belly fat genes and frying flab—and that's on top of all their other health-boosting benefits.

These powerful veggies remind us a bit of those overachievers you loved to hate in high school—you know, the ones who not only got straight A's but also scored the hottest date to prom and got voted soccer captain, too. The primary difference between produce and Mr. Popular? Veggies don't aim to make you jealous with their superhuman skills, they want you to use them to your advantage so you can reach your better body goals.

PEPPERS

You may have heard that spicy hot peppers can help you scorch calories, but did you know that mild peppers can have the same effect? Thanks to a metabolism-boosting compound, dihydrocapsiate, and their high vitamin-C content, sweet red and green peppers can help you lose weight. A cup of these bell-shaped veggies serves up to three times the day's recommended vitamin C—a nutrient that counteracts stress hormones which trigger fat storage around the midsection. Dip slices of bell peppers into hummus for a light afternoon snack, add the veggie to omelets and salads, or throw some chicken in a corn tortilla with salsa and slices of avocado, red pepper and onion for a Tex-Mex-inspired fat-fighting dinner.

BROCCOLI

In addition to warding off prostate, breast, lung and skin cancers, this flowery vegetable can also help you whittle your middle. According to experts, broccoli contains a phytonutrient called sulforaphane that increase testosterone and fights off body fat storage. It's also rich in vitamin C (a mere cup of the stuff can help you hit your daily mark), a nutrient that can lower levels of cortisol during stressful situations, helping those abs take center stage. The only downside? It can make some people with sensitive stomachs a bit gassy—which isn't a good look if you're planning to hit the beach or rock a tight-fitting outfit. That's no reason to steer clear of this veggie on a day-to-day basis, though. Whip up our Garlicky Beef and Broccoli with Broccoli Noodles recipe to reap the belly-flattening benefits —just not the day before you need to look your leanest.

SPINACH

It may look pretty unassuming, but Popeye's favorite veggie can actually help take your calorie-burning potential to the next level. How? The green is overflowing with protein (just one cup of the steamed variety has as much protein as a medium hard-boiled egg), a nutrient that aids post-pump muscle recovery and growth. And remember; the more muscle mass you have, the more calories you burn at rest! What's more, the leafy green is also rich in thylakoids, a compound that's been shown to significantly reduce cravings and promote weight loss. Add the green to your dinner plate to reap the benefits. We like to steam it and flavor it with garlic, olive oil and lemon.

PICKLES

Pickles are low-cal, filled with fiber and covered in vinegar—which is all good news for your waistline. In fact, just one large pickle has 15 calories and 2 grams of belly-filling fiber, so eating three or four can actually leave you feeling pretty satiated for less than 100 calories! Every dieter knows that eating filling snacks are paramount to weight-loss success, but how does the vinegar help the fat-fighting cause? Studies shows acidic foods help increase the rate at which the body burns off carbs by up to 40 percent—and the faster you burn off carbs, the sooner your body starts incinerating fat, which can help you get that lean look you crave. Add these tangy, pickled cucumbers to sandwiches and burgers or munch on them solo to start feeling more confident in your skivvies.

POTATOES

If you typically eat your potatoes warm out of the oven, you're missing out on the spud's fat-fighting superpowers. When you throw potatoes in the refrigerator and eat them cold, their digestible starches turn into resistant starches through a process called retrogradation. As the name implies, resistant starch, well, resists digestion, which promotes fat oxidation and reduces abdominal fat. Since eating cold baked potatoes don't sound too appetizing, why not use the cooled spuds to make a potato salad instead? Here's how: Bake red potatoes in the oven until they're cooked through and allow them to fully cool. Then cut them into small slices and dress them with Dijon mustard, fresh pepper, chopped green onions (more on this veggie next), dill and plain Greek yogurt. Mix everything together and put in the refrigerator to cool before consuming.

ONIONS

Onions are rich in quercetin, a flavonoid that increase blood flow and activates a protein in the body that helps regulate glucose levels, torches stored fat and keeps new fat cells from forming. Not to mention, onions are basically the unsung hero of cardiovascular health—an important area of wellness for everyone, but especially those who hit the gym hard to accelerate their weight-loss efforts. The culinary staple can help lower cholesterol, ward off hardening of the arteries and help maintain healthy blood-pressure levels. The best part? Onions are super low-cal and easy to throw into just about anything, from soups, homemade burgers, sandwiches and tacos to pastas, salads, veggie sides, rice and omelets.

SUPER FRUITS

We have combed through the listings to give you some of the best fruits that will aid in weight loss process. Most of the fruits that will be mentioned in this article have already won raves for their ability to do wonders on your body's weight, but there will be others you never knew had such effect on your weight. These fruits are wholesome in themselves thereby curbing any unnecessary craving you develop. In today's world where health is not always wealth, this article will serve you some pointers that you will need to bear in mind for healthy lifestyle. Read below to get a list of power fruits to be taken in moderation that will do the trick to your health and weight.

Best Fruits For Weight Loss

AVOCADO:

This is the first fruit to top the list and that too for a reason. It's simple. Because it is the best fruit for weight loss.

Avocado is enriched with omega 9 fatty acids and is a great way to lose weight. It speeds up metabolism by burning the fat and boosting energy. You will also derive several other health benefits. So have an avocado on a regular basis and you will lose weight and stay fit. So make a salad or guacamole and the difference will be visible.

LEMON:

You can never find a combination unlike lemon and honey that will marvellously help you lose weight. Lemon is a weight management fruit that has wallops of riboflavin, Vitamin B, minerals like phosphorus and magnesium, not to mention Vitamin C. Drink a concoction of lemon and honey every morning and there's no better way to start your day than with this detoxifier.

WATERMELON:

This fruit requires a special mention because it is devoid of any fat. The maximum calories you can squeeze out of it when you consume one glass of watermelon juice is 50 calories. Also, it is rich in Vitamins A, B and C and packed full of the plant chemical, lycopene, which will protect you against heart diseases and cancer.

BANANAS:

This fruit is best taken in the raw and green state as it contains more soluble starch. Consumption of one banana will give you a full stomach and sipping a little water after this will help you stave off any cravings. It will provide you with the requisite energy your body needs as it burns fat more quickly.

GRAPEFRUIT:

Recent studies have shown that people consuming grapefruit on a daily basis tend to lose much more weight than if they don't do so. Grape is a high carbohydrate fruit that is best taken as part of your breakfast because it can compensate for the night's fasting with its high sugar content and will also help in the day's digestive process for your body.

ORANGE:

If you are worried about munching on to something, then go for oranges. High in water content and low in calories, this fruit will satiate your emotional hunger and will help lose weight. So that's two birds with one stone.

APPLE:

Any plans for controlling the food intake in between meals? Then grab an apple as it will not only keep the doctor away but also being high in fiber, Vitamin A and water content, it's going to give you that fullness in your stomach.

POMEGRANATE:

Grace yourself with pomegranate seeds as it deserves all the attention it garners in the nutrition world. Its seeds are rich in antioxidants, fibres, and water content. What more? They are low in calories, so chew a couple of this pomegranate seeds and it will not sabotage your diet.

PINEAPPLE:

What is the deal with pineapples and weight loss? Pineapples are rich in antioxidants, enzymes, minerals, vitamins and you name it. But what helps it lose weight? Well, it's the fact that this fruit is free of cholesterol and fat.

BERRIES:

Blueberries, strawberries, raspberries, cranberries etc are citrus fruits that will impart very little carbohydrates to your body. But they play excellent detoxifiers and bowel cleansers. They will not only aid digestion but will also take the spotlight in weight loss.

These are the top fruits that help in weight loss!

SUPER COMPLEX CARBOHYDRATES

Most people decide to go on a diet and immediately eliminate carbohydrates. However, while white bread, white pasta, and baked goods with white refined flour might sabotage your weight loss efforts; all carbs can't be painted with the same red brush.

Carbohydrates don't make you fat.

In fact, if you cut carbs completely out of your diet, sure you'd be eliminating many starchy foods, but you'd also be eliminating fruits, vegetables, and whole grains, resulting in serious food cravings that would send you on a supersized binge at the nearest drive-thru burger joint—STAT!

Carbohydrates are essential for energy and brain function, and if you consume the following ten nutrient-dense, fiber-rich carbs, you'll stay fueled, lose weight, and stay full all day long…

Oatmeal

Oatmeal is high in soluble fiber, which means that it dissolves slowly after you eating, keeping you sustained for much longer than, say, crispy rice cereal. Plus, food studies link oatmeal to blasting visceral fat, which is the hard to combat fat that sits around your mid-section and your vital organs (i.e., your heart).

Bulgur Wheat

Bulgur wheat, or more precisely, cracked wheat, is a tad time-consuming to prepare—it needs to be soaked in hot water before boiling. However, the effort to make up a batch for a week of dinners will seem miniscule when you consider that this fiber-rich grain packs 5-grams of slow-burning fiber in just a half cup!

Beans

Beans, beans are good for your heart! And yes, the more you eat; the more regular your digestive system will function, which aids greatly in weight loss. Plus, in addition to being high in fiber, beans also pack valuable amounts of protein and iron to fuel your workouts.

Wheat Berries

Wheat berries are getting more attention lately. Once relegated to vegetarians and health food aficionados, these mini kernels of whole wheat pack plenty of fiber, iron, magnesium, zinc, and B vitamins, which help the transfer food into energy and boost metabolic rate (calorie to fuel production).

Quinoa

Quinoa isn't considered a "super food" without merit. Quinoa is a super protein, meaning it contains the essential amino acids needed to build lean muscle and rev up your metabolic rate (the speed at which you burn calories). So in addition to eating a grain that's packed with protein, quinoa doesn't contain the harmful fat that meat does.

SUPER DAIRY

Keeping a food diary is a great way to take a look at your eating habits including what you eat, when you eat, and how you feel when you eat. It can also help you identify possible food intolerances, and if your goal happens to include losing a few pounds, a food log is a great weight-loss tool. In fact, starting a food diary is often the first thing registered dietitians ask their clients to do. The simple act of writing down what you eat can help increase self-awareness, which may lead you to make healthier choices.

In order to make sure you're getting the most out of creating a food diary you want to make sure you're keeping tabs on the right things.

Here are the six food logging.

Set up a method that works for you.

Take your lifestyle into consideration, "There are many online tools, apps, and handwritten versions of food journals and trackers that can be quite helpful." try jotting your food down in a note on your phone or using a good old-fashioned notebook.

If you're a visual person, a photo food journal is another good option. "I say focus on making calories count instead of just counting calories alone Look for a variety of food groups and colors, and pay attention to portion sizes."

Consider recording times and emotions, too.

If you're setting up your own food journal (instead of using an app), there are few details you'll want to write down. "The key elements for documentation are spaces for breakfast, lunch, and dinner, plus two to three spaces for snacks, a space for exercise, and a space for behavior or feeling.

Recording the time you eat can also be helpful—personally, when I started logging my food, I noticed that most of my mindless snacking happened after dinner. After recognizing that, I started eating more filling dinners with protein and fiber to keep me full and away from the munchies in my cupboard.

Start by writing things down as you eat them.

"Make a commitment to log items right after you eat them," suggests Pine. "If you wait until the end of the day, you're probably more likely to forget accurate portion sizes and not include small tastes of food, beverages, and condiments." Plus, after a crazy day at the office or running around, logging everything you ate that day can just feel too overwhelming to bother with.

And vow to be completely honest with yourself.

"If you aren't honest with a food journal, the only person you're hurting is yourself," Even though it's tempting to only log the good stuff, hold yourself accountable for writing it all down—even the things you're not thrilled with. Record 100 percent of what you eat— every beverage and every little nibble (even from someone else's plate) needs to be accounted for."

"Making dinner and tasting your dish while cooking? Write it down. At work and passing the candy bowl for just one piece? Write it down"We do a lot of mindless eating that we don't always account for. Writing it down is a very visual way of seeing your habits."

Don't get too caught up in the calories (but be aware of them).

"While starting a food diary is a fantastic way to become more aware of the food we are eating, it is important to keep in mind that calories are not the only thing that matters when it comes to good nutrition. "Sure, counting calories can help give you a more accurate picture of what you're consuming, but a 1,500-calorie diet full of processed food is much, much different than a 1,500-calorie diet full of fresh fruits, vegetables, and whole grains."

Plus, while calorie counting can give you a good estimate of what foods you're overeating (even healthy but high-calorie ones, like avocados or almonds), it's impossible to be entirely sure. "My number one-piece of advice when starting a food diary is not to look for perfection, as you will never be able to 100 percent accurately track your intake, so watch out for becoming obsessed with calories.

Most importantly, use your food log to learn about your eating habits.

"A food journal may initially tell you how many calories or grams of sugar and fat you are eating, but it can tell you so much more. Food diaries are not meant to make you feel bad, but rather to make you aware of your choices and eating habits. They give you insight to your relationship with food."

And it's not all about seeing where you can improve—take notice of the things you're proud of, too. "Look for things you are doing well and pat yourself on the back for those things in addition to the things you can improve upon.

When approached in a healthy and mindful way, food logs can be a great way to jumpstart weight loss and get to know yourself a little better in the process. Plus, it's a great excuse to invest in a pretty new notebook, right?

Greek Yogurt

Its tangy taste and creamy texture makes Greek yogurt an appealing option to yogurt enthusiasts. While Greek yogurt has no special weight loss powers, as a higher source of satiating protein than regular yogurt, the Mediterranean-style yogurt may be a better choice for those on a weight-loss diet. If you're trying to drop a few pounds, consider working Greek yogurt to your diet.

Greek Yogurt Nutrition Basics

When weight loss is your goal, use non-fat Greek yogurt to get the most benefits without the extra calories. A 6-ounce container of plain, nonfat Greek yogurt has 100 calories, 17 grams of protein and 6 grams of carbs. While plain, nonfat regular yogurt has fewer calories, it is higher in carbs and lower in protein. The same serving of regular yogurt has 95 calories, 10 grams of protein and 13 grams of carbs.

Protein and Weight Loss

Although plain, non-fat Greek yogurt is a little higher in calories than the regular non-fat yogurt, you might gain more benefits from its higher protein content when you're trying to lose weight than merely saving those 5 calories. Getting a higher percentage of your calories from protein -- as much as 30 percent -- according to to a 2015 study published in Food Science and Nutrition, offers a number of benefits when it comes to weight loss, including better hunger control, preservation of muscle mass and an increase in your calorie-burning power.

Greek Yogurt for Weight Loss

In addition, an increase in dairy foods, such as Greek yogurt, are also associated with weight loss. A 2005 study published in the International Journal of Obesity investigated the effects of a calorie-reduced diet with and without yogurt on weight loss in a group of obese people. The researchers found that the yogurt-eating group lost more weight than the non-yogurt eating group. However, it's important to note that the yogurt used in the study was regular non-fat yogurt, not Greek yogurt. Clinical studies using the higher-protein yogurt are necessary before claims can be made. The study also included regular exercise, which is an important aspect of any weight loss program.

WHAT ABOUT CALCIUM?

In addition to protein, there's also a significant difference in calcium content between Greek and regular yogurt. This is an important distinction, because it is also thought that the calcium in dairy foods may be partly responsible for the weight loss benefits of dairy foods. A 6-ounce container of plain nonfat Greek yogurt contains 110 milligrams of calcium, while the same serving of plain non-fat regular yogurt contains 338 milligrams. Even though it is lower in calcium than regular yogurt, Greek yogurt still fits well in a weight-loss diet. Just make sure you're getting enough other high-calcium foods -- such as milk, cheese or fortified foods -- to meet your daily calcium needs. For reference, adults need 1,000 milligrams to 1,200 milligrams of calcium a day.

Tips and Servings

Greek yogurt makes a healthy addition to any weight-loss diet. It's filling, high in protein, yet low in calories and a good source of calcium. Buy the plain variety and add fresh fruit to bump up the nutrition. The tangy yogurt also makes a healthy topper for your baked potato or you can use it to increase the protein content in a fruit smoothie.

What's important to keep in mind when it comes to weight loss is your overall calorie intake. Even if all your calories come from healthy sources, such as non-fat Greek yogurt, eating more than your body needs will result in weight gain, not loss.

CONCLUSION

Weight control methods can be successful if weight loss dieting is maintained without compromising overall health. When you get successful in weight reduction program, you also promote permanent life-style changes. The physical and psychological benefits of maintaining the right weight can be observed when it is done the right way. It is, however, more beneficial when you personalize the weight reduction plan based on individual needs and lifestyle.

When you get the right ingredients of weight loss dieting like exercise and sleep, you tend to get the weight you desire. We know that getting the right weight also prevents us from certain diseases. Not only that, we function well in our daily workload. We become successful when we do our job right. For all of us, it is definitely important that we look good. By getting the proper nutrition and understanding how the body works, we get the optimum level of health and it gives you the glow you deserve. Sometimes, we just overlook the secrets of getting the best of us. We fail to identify how we get through with getting healthy and looking good. Therefore, being conscious about our weight and our physical appearance is not bad at all. It actually reflects on how we live our lives and how we become effective creatures. Being healthy gives you an overall good functionality.

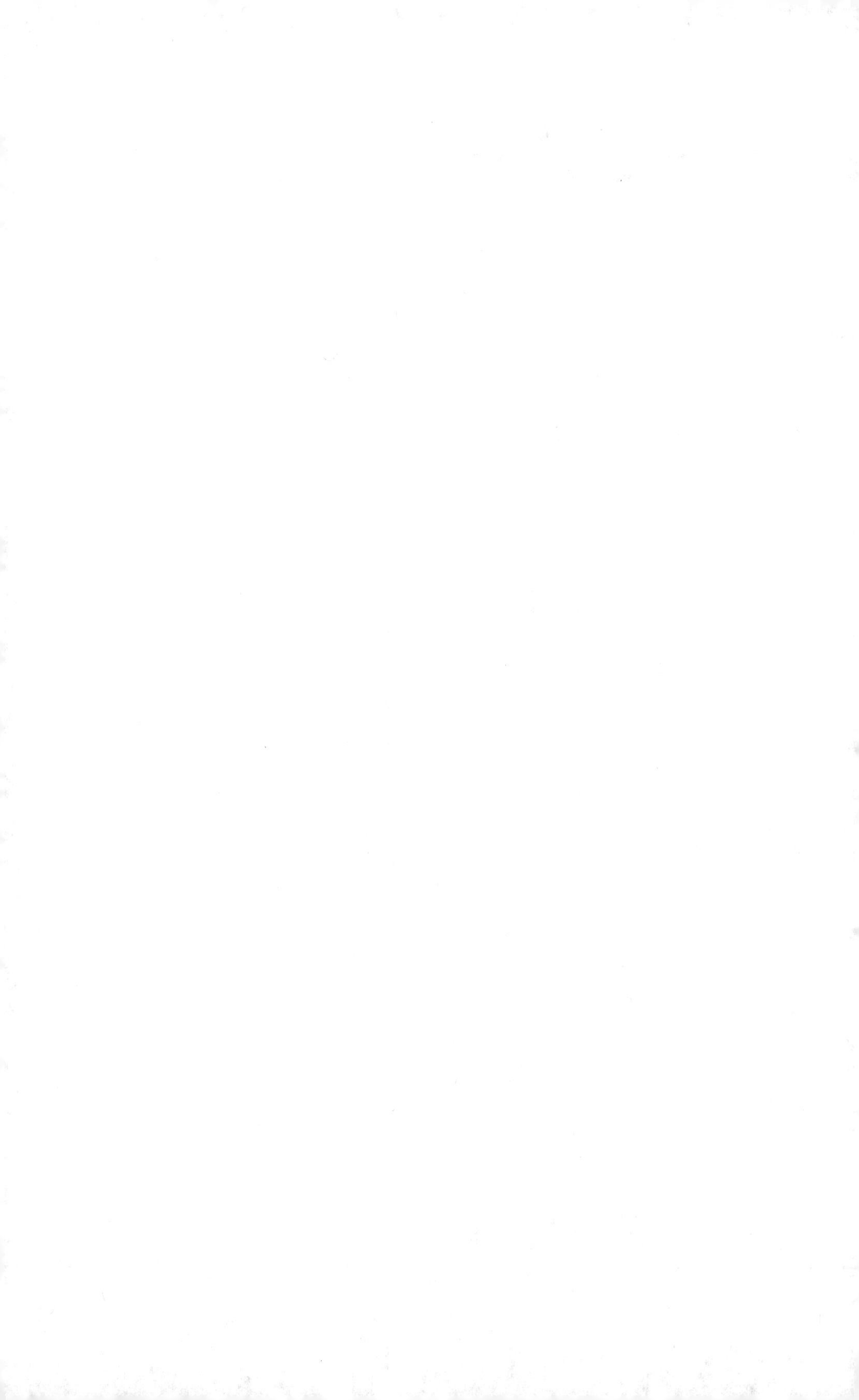